Balance Exercises
for Seniors

Balance Exercises for Seniors

Easy to Perform Fall Prevention Workouts to Improve Stability and Posture

BAZ THOMPSON

Contents

Introduction xi

Benefits of Exercise xii

Types of Exercise xiv

Exercises in this Book xv

How to Use This Book xvi

01 THE IMPORTANCE OF BALANCE 1

The Science of Balance 1

Fear of Falling 3

Test Your Balance 6

02 SEATED EXERCISES 9

Forward Punch 10

Hip Abduction Side Kick 11

Hip External Rotator Stretch 12

Hip Flexion Fold 13

Isometric Back Extensor Hold 14

Lateral Trunk Flexion 15

Seated Marching 16

Sit-to-Stand 17

Toe Raises 18

Trunk Circles 19

03   STANDING EXERCISES 21

3-Way Hip Kick 23

Foot Taps 24

Heel Raises 25

Lateral Stepping 26

Mini Lunges 27

Narrow Stance Reach 28

Single Leg Stance 29

Squats 30

Standing Marches 31

Tandem Stance 32

04   WALKING EXERCISES 33

Backward Walking 35

Balance Walking 36

Ball Toss 37

Curb Walking 38

Dynamic Walking 39

Grapevine 40

Heel-to-Toe 41

Side Steps 42

Walk on Heels and Toes 43

Zigzag Walking 44

05   CORE EXERCISES 45

Bridge 47

Forearm Plank 48

Modified Plank. 49

Opposite Arm and Leg Raise. 50

Seated Forward Roll Up 51

Seated Half Roll-Backs 52

Seated Leg Lifts 53

Seated Leg Taps 54

Seated Side Bends. 55

Superman 56

06 Vestibular Exercises 57

Eyes Side-to-Side. 58

Eyes Up and Down 59

Gaze Stabilization Sitting 60

Gaze Stabilization Standing 61

Head and Eyes Opposite Direction. 62

Head and Eyes Same Direction 63

Head Bend. 64

Head Turn. 65

Shoulder Turns. 66

Smooth Pursuits. 67

07 Exercise Routines 69

Core Focus Week 70

Leg Strength Week. 71

Brain Training Week 72

Walking and Movement Week. 73

Conclusion 75

References 79

BEFORE YOU
START READING

As a special gift, I included a logbook and my book, "**Strength Training After 40**" (regularly priced at $16.97 on Amazon) and the best part is, you get access to all of them for **FREE**.

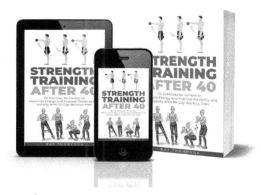

What's in it for me?

○ 101 highly effective strength training exercises that can help you reach the highest point of your fitness performance

○ Foundational exercises to improve posture and increase range of motion in your arms, shoulders, chest, and back

○ Stretches to help you gain flexibility and find deep relaxation

SCAN THE QR CODE

Workout Logbook to help you keep track of your accomplishments and progress. Log your progress to give you the edge you need to accomplish your goals.

Introduction

Aging is not lost youth but a new stage of opportunity and strength.

Betty Freidan

Welcome to the initial step in regaining and maintaining your balance! You may be currently having stability issues, recovering from an injury, or just taking preventative steps to keep physically strong and well balanced. We will walk on this journey together to learn about our bodies, discover how to stay strong and stable as our bodies age, and employ simple steps to keep, or recover, our balance.

The Vestibular Disorders Association defines balance this way:

> Balance is the ability to maintain the body's center of mass over its base of support. A properly functioning balance system allows humans to see clearly while moving, identify orientation with respect to gravity, determine direction and speed of movement, and make automatic postural adjustments to maintain posture and stability in various conditions and activities. (Watson, et al., n.d.).

In other words, balance is the capability to remain stable and upright. When we think of balance, certain things come to mind, such as: a person learning to ride a unicycle, a young gymnast walking on a balance beam, or a trapeze artist walking on a tightrope. These activities all involve a good deal of balance and may be things some people are not ever able to do. But balance is more than circus tricks and gymnastic feats. It is an important and vital part of functioning in our everyday lives. Some ways that we use balance in our daily life include:

- ○ Getting up out of bed

- ○ Walking across the room

- ○ Sitting down in a chair

- ○ Going up and down stairs

- ○ Getting in and out of cars

- ○ Carrying bags and packages

- ○ Turning to look behind you

- ○ Stepping aside to let others pass you

- ○ Reaching forward to grasp something

Our body's natural ability to balance starts to slowly diminish once we reach our mid-40's. As we age, things that contribute to the decline in balance include vision problems, inner ear issues, and other injuries or illnesses. One of the overlooked causes of the loss of balance, however, is inactivity. When older adults become sedentary and lose muscular strength in their core, upper body, and lower body, a loss of balance follows. The good news is balance can be regained and maintained with regular exercise and training. All ages can improve their balance and become stronger, but those who are over 40 years old should incorporate balance exercises into their regular activity routine.

BENEFITS OF EXERCISE

Balance exercises ought to be done regularly, along with cardio, weights, and stretching, as part of a fitness and preventative program. Why exercise? We all know that regular exercise is good for you, but it is especially important as we age. The Surgeon General reports that as we age, we become less active. A third of all men and half of all women engage in no physical activity by the time they are 75 years old (CDC, 2019). This reduced activity leads to a loss of stamina and strength.

Misconceptions

First, some misconceptions about exercise should be addressed. Perhaps you have heard people say these or have even thought about them yourself. Common misconceptions about exercise include:

1. **I'm too old.** If you are still alive, you aren't too old to start an exercise program. Older adults who have either never exercised or are just getting back into exercising again after years of inactivity quickly show improvement in their physical and mental capacities by participating in regular movement and exertion.

2. **I'm not the athlete I was.** For those who were very active or competitive athletes in their youth, it can be disheartening to not have the ability or strength to do what they once were able to do. By remembering that we all are getting older, we can be realistic about expectations. Our bodies change over time and certain abilities decline with age, but a sense of satisfaction and enjoyment can still be had by participating in age-appropriate activities.

3. **I will get old anyway.** Exercise doesn't stop us from getting older, but it does help us look and feel younger. Regular physical activity boosts energy, helps maintain or lose weight, and bolsters the immune system. By staying healthy, we get to enjoy longer life and stay independent while living it.

4. **I'm disabled or in ill health.** If this is your situation, you have extra challenges in getting movement into your life. However, starting off slowly and gently with what you are able to do, such as stretching or other gentle activities like chair yoga, can get you on a path that eventually will allow you to do more as you get stronger. Getting in some type of consistent and gentle physical activity will also help you manage aches and pains better.

Advantages of Exercise

There are advantages to starting and keeping consistent with an exercise plan. The specific benefits that come from exercising include:

1. **Prevention of disease.** Exercise boosts the immune system of the body and helps ward off illnesses such as colds and flus, but it also can help prevent more serious conditions such as heart disease, high blood pressure, and diabetes. Physical activity such as walking, swimming, and biking are all good ways to get moving. Activities such as bowling, dancing, tennis, and golf are some non-impact sports that are suitable for aging adults.

2. **Promotion of good mental health.** Exercise and prolonged activities cause the body to produce the feel-good hormones called endorphins. When released into our body systems, these hormones relieve stress and promote a sense of happiness and well-being. Getting in some physical activity also results in better and deeper sleep at night. Many older adults have trouble sleeping, sometimes because of inactivity.

3. **Improvement of cognitive function.** Because physical activity requires the use of large, small, and fine motor skills, it stimulates cognitive functioning in the brain. The risk of dementia and other age-related decline in cognitive abilities increases as we age but the likelihood of it happening can be reduced with regular exercise.

4. **Lessened fall risks.** Older adults take longer to recover from injuries resulting from a fall, and that can lead to a loss of independence. Exercise increases the body's strength, agility, and flexibility, all of which are needed to help prevent falls.

5. **Engagement with others.** Maintaining ties to groups of friends or the local community is important as we age to help prevent isolation as well as feelings of depression and loneliness. By exercising at a gym or with others, we can make physical exercise a fun and social activity.

TYPES OF EXERCISE

Finding a form of physical activity that you enjoy is a key component to maintaining consistency in the long-term. Exercise does not need to be strenuous to be effective. Spending hours at the gym on the treadmill or lifting heavy weights is not realistic or helpful once we hit the senior years. But some type of physical exertion is important and should be done daily or at least five days a week, according to the U.S. Department of Health and Human Services (Elsawy and Higgens, 2010).

The areas of exercise that ought to be included are:

○ **Cardiovascular.** Sometimes simply called cardio, this type of exercise uses the large muscle groups in your body and elevates the heart rate. Practiced regularly, it lessens fatigue and decreases shortness of breath along with strengthening the heart.

- Examples include: cycling, dancing, hiking, rowing, stair climbing, swimming, tennis, and walking.

- Recommended time: 150 minutes of moderate-intensity aerobic activity (30 minutes, five days a week) or 75 minutes of vigorous-intensity aerobic activity (20 minutes, five days a week).

○ **Strength Training.** This type of exercise involves lifting or pushing against something with resistance. The repetitive motion and resistance helps to build bone mass, muscle, and strength.

- Examples include: hand held or free weights, weight machines, resistance bands, or your own body weight.

- Recommended time: strength training of all the major muscle groups two days a week.

○ **Flexibility.** Keeping your muscles and joints limber and able to move freely through a full range of motion is the goal of flexibility exercises. It has been said that "motion is lotion" when it comes to joint health.

- Examples include: calisthenics, yoga, tai chi, and stretching.
- Recommended time: 10 minutes, two days a week.

○ **Balance Exercises.** Starting in our mid-40's, our balance abilities start to slowly decline. However, practicing and training our balance with regular exercises can help regain and maintain our equilibrium and stability.

- Examples include: seated exercises, standing exercises, walking, core exercises, and vestibular exercises that all target balance and strength.
- Recommended time: 10 minutes, five days a week.

EXERCISES IN THIS BOOK

For the remainder of this book, we will be concentrating on the last type of exercise; balance exercises. The goal is to inform you, the reader, on the whys and hows of balance exercises as well as give you 50 exercises that you can start doing today to work on your equilibrium and stability. It is never too early, or too late, to start building your ability to balance.

○ In Chapter 1, we will take a look at how our brain keeps our body in balance as well as some statistics on losing your balance and what the results of that are long-term. We will also talk about the risk factors for falls and how to reduce them. At the end of the chapter, there is a list of balance tests for you to perform to gauge how you are doing in terms of balance.

○ Chapter 2 concentrates on seated balance exercises. These exercises only require a sturdy chair and will work on building stability from a seated position.

○ Standing balance exercises are outlined in Chapter 3. Working on strength and steadiness while in a standing position is what we focus on in this chapter.

○ In Chapter 4, we will take a look at adding movement in with some standing balance exercises. These walking exercises require some multitasking and will help build confidence in your ability to balance while walking.

- ○ Chapter 5 targets core strength. Our abdominal and back muscles are key to our overall capacity for good balance, so we will spotlight the ways we can build power in our core.

- ○ The vestibular system is addressed in Chapter 6. We focus here on exercises that retrain our brain, eyes, and inner ear for good equilibrium.

- ○ In Chapter 7, we include some tailored workout routines that incorporate the exercises found in the previous chapters. It is a good starting point for a month's worth of weekly routines that include core strength, leg strength, vestibular strength, and walking.

HOW TO USE THIS BOOK

Not only will you learn important information about your body and the subject of balance, you will also find 50 practical exercises that you can start using right away. Look at this book as a balance guidebook that you can refer back to again and again.

In each of the chapters containing exercises, the individual moves will include the amount of time each exercise takes to complete, the areas of the body that you are working on, and detailed directions on how to do the exercise. Many exercises will include instructions on how to take the move to the next level and make it more challenging once you have gotten stronger and more stable. At the end of each exercise will be reminders on what to take note of and cautions to remember. Illustrations that accompany each exercise will show each move done correctly, and will guide you and help you to position your head, body, arms, legs, and feet accordingly. As mentioned previously, you can work through each exercise in this book, one at a time, or follow the exercise plans that are included towards the end of the book. Find a way for these exercises to work for you, then stick with it. You can achieve better balance and equilibrium with some effort!

If you are starting any new type of activity, you are encouraged to consult with your doctor prior to embarking on any exercise program.

Getting older is inevitable for us all, but losing our balance and experiencing falls do not have to go along with aging. By becoming educated on our bodies, learning to make the changes we need to, deciding to take steps to better health, and then finally following through with our decisions with action, we can all enjoy the second half of our lives with good health and vitality.

Thank you so much for downloading my book. I would love to hear your thoughts so be sure to leave a review on Amazon. This will help many other people who are in the same situation as you find my book. It would mean a lot to me.

SCAN THE QR CODE

My hope and goal is that you will find this book a helpful tool as you work on regaining and maintaining good balance to prevent falls and enhance your overall well being. Are you ready? Let's get your fitness education and training started!

THE IMPORTANCE OF BALANCE

Getting old is like climbing a mountain; you get a little out of breath, but the view is much better!

~ Ingmar Bergman

It has been said that aging is not for the faint of heart. If we consider the importance of balance, we could add that aging is also not for those who lose their balance. Remaining strong and stable is crucial to living a vibrant and active life as you approach your 60s, 70s, 80s, and beyond. Balance and stability in our bodies helps us to maintain our physical health and do the things we enjoy.

What happens, however, when we have a loss in the ability to keep our good balance? In this chapter, we will learn about the three body systems that contribute to our balance. We will also look at the biggest consequence when we no longer have good balance, what increases our risks for falling, and what can be done to prevent it. We will also learn how to test our balance at home.

THE SCIENCE OF BALANCE

Mike was a car enthusiast who enjoyed taking his vintage convertible out for a drive every Sunday. Sometimes, he would take along one of his grandkids and they would stop for ice cream. The convertible was parked in his extra car garage. To get there, Mike would walk from his concrete driveway, across the grass in his side yard, and onto a gravel path. Although he was in his late sixties, Mike didn't have any problems transitioning from one walking surface to the next because he had good balance and a stable core. His Aston-Martin was sleek, fast, and sat low to the ground, making it a fun car to drive with the top down. Mike easily got in and out of the driver's seat because his legs and core were strong.

It is easy to take good balance for granted. But someone with impaired balance would have had a difficult time in the scenario above. Stumbling over surface transitions and having trouble squatting up and down into a lowered seat can be tiring and even dangerous for a person who struggles with balance issues.

The Hows of Balance

How does our body maintain balance and equilibrium? There are three main body systems that contribute to our overall balance. These include sensory input from three areas of our bodies, the processing of that input, and our bodies reaction to the input.

Sensory Input

Our brains receive information from all parts of our bodies. For balance, the brain particularly looks at the nerve impulses received from the eyes, the ears, and the muscles and joints in our arms and legs.

- **Visual.** The rods and cones in our eyes send messages to the the brain to help it determine where our bodies are in relation to our surroundings. These visual cues help us to approach or avoid things in our path and keep us aligned.

- **Touch.** Sensors in our skin, muscles, and joints relay information so that our brain knows when we are taking a step forward, which way our head is turned, and where our body is in the space we are occupying.

- **Vestibular.** The inner canals and working of our ears make up the majority of the vestibular system. It contributes to the awareness of equilibrium and motion. The impulses that the sensors send to the brain allows us to know if we are standing, lying down, or turning, among other things.

Integration of Input

The coming together of all the input received in the brain is broken down and assigned to certain parts of the brain. The brain stem combines and sorts information from the senses.

- **Cerebellum.** Called the coordination center of the brain, the cerebellum regulates posture and balance. It relies on automatic reactions and previous

2

history from repeated exposure to certain actions. This is the part of the brain that helps a racquetball player know what kind of balance they will need to serve the ball.

○ **Cerebral cortex.** This thinking and memory command center of the brain contributes to memory and critical thinking, like decision making. Stored information in this area helps a person remember that walking on a rainy street requires extra caution because of slip hazards and slick surfaces.

Motor Input

Finally, the brain stem again comes into the picture. It sends messages to all areas of the body and tells it what to do to maintain balance. Some reflexes include:

○ **Eye reflex.** Called the vestibulo-ocular reflex, this automatic function of our eyes is triggered by the information coming from the brain. It allows your gaze to remain steady, even if your head is moving from side to side or up and down.

○ **Motor impulses.** These oversee eye movements and make body adjustments. With the information from the brain, your muscles and joints can move in the way they need to based on information from your eyes. If you have ever seen a dancer or ice skater twirl around and around repeatedly while keeping their balance, you have seen this motor impulse in action.

FEAR OF FALLING

Marilyn was a mother and grandmother who loved to spend time with her kids and grandchildren on a regular basis. She loved to bake with her grandkids and take them to the movies. At one time, Marilyn was an avid tennis player, but because she was now in her early seventies, she didn't play as much tennis as she used to. She also didn't feel like going to the gym anymore because the exercise classes were just too hard for her. Her joints became more creaky and her arthritis flared up from time to time, but overall she was doing okay. She was in the kitchen one day, reaching for a baking pan that was at the back of the shelf, when she lost her balance and fell. As she was falling, she hit her head on the edge of the countertop before landing on her hip on the kitchen tile flooring. She wound up with stitches for the cut on her forehead and a broken hip that required surgery. Because of the injuries she sustained, Marilyn not only lost her mobility, but lost some of her independence to drive and get around on her own as well.

Falls are not a normal part of aging. Yet, every year, millions of older adults lose their balance, fall, and injure themselves. The Center for Disease Control (CDC) statistics related to falls are sobering. They include:

- One-fourth of adults over 65 years old fall each year.

- Once you fall, your chance for falling again doubles.

- Emergency rooms across the nation see over three million older adults for injuries related to falls and 800,000 of those are hospitalized because of head or hip injuries that are a result from their fall.

- One-fifth of falls cause serious injury like head trauma or broken bones.

- Traumatic brain injuries are most commonly caused by a fall.

- Over 95 percent of hip fractures are the result of a fall (CDC, 2019).

While falls may not always cause serious injury, twenty percent of the time, the injuries are bad enough that it becomes difficult for the injured person to accomplish everyday activities, drive, or live independently.

Fall Risk Factors

While anyone can accidentally trip and fall, there are certain conditions that make it more likely for you to fall. These risk factors include:

- **Vision problems.** Because of age and either injury or illness, we can experience problems with our vision. Not being able to see objects at our feet or in our pathway can cause us to stumble over them and potentially fall.

- **Foot pain.** Having foot pain can occur from either injury to the foot or simply from ill-fitting shoes that lack support and grip. To maintain balance, we need the sensory feedback from our feet, ankles, knees, and hips.

- **Prescription and over-the-counter medications.** Doctor prescribed medications can sometimes cause dizziness or drowsiness, especially pain medication, sedatives, tranquilizers, and antidepressants. OTC medications such as antihistamines, cough syrups, and cold medicines can also affect your steadiness on your feet.

- **Vitamin D deficiency.** The relationship between vitamin D and good bone health is well established. There is also some evidence that when vitamin D levels fall below a certain point in the body, muscle functioning is decreased and the risk for falls increases (Akdeniz et al., 2016).

- **Trip hazards in the home.** Uneven steps, loose carpeting or floor tiles, electrical cords, and throw rugs are all common trip hazards at home. Poor or dim lighting, items left on the floor, and water or other liquid that has spilled on the floor are other dangers that can contribute to falls.

○ **Core and lower body weakness.** Older adults can sometimes become fearful of falling and cut back on their physical activities. Unfortunately, the old saying "if you don't use it, you lose it" is true when it comes to core and leg strength. Less stamina and strength in the lower half of the body is a contributing factor in the occurrence of falls.

Four Ways to Prevent Falls

Now that we know what can contribute to falls as we grow older, we are going to take a look at how we can be proactive and prevent falls from happening. Remember, falling is not a normal part of aging! It is avoidable with just a few preemptive steps, such as:

○ **Have your eyes and feet examined.** The doctor will not only look at the overall health of your eyesight, but can prescribe an updated prescription for glasses or contacts as well. Clear vision is necessary to avoid falls. Have your healthcare provider look at your feet and the shoes you normally wear, and get a recommendation for a podiatrist if necessary.

○ **Get an annual checkup.** Every year, get an assessment of your health from your general practitioner or healthcare provider. Talk with your doctor about any dizziness or balance issues that you have had and have them review the list of prescription medications you take to see if there are any interactions that may contribute to feelings of dizziness, drowsiness, or instability. Ask about vitamin D supplements that can improve your bone and muscle health.

○ **Make your home trip-proof.** Clear all the walking areas of your home from any clutter, books, or small objects that you can potentially fall over. Remove scatter rugs or tape them down securely with double-sided rug tape. Use non-slip mats in the bathroom and other areas that have tile flooring. Keep commonly used items in easy-to-reach places to avoid using step stools or ladders. Assess the lighting in your home and switch out lamps or bulbs for ones that offer clear, warm lights to help you see better.

○ **Maintain a regular fitness program.** Discuss with your doctor or a physical trainer how you can exercise safely and incorporate cardiovascular, strength training, flexibility, and balance exercises into a daily routine. As you gain strength, stamina, and confidence, you decrease your chances of falling and injuring yourself.

TEST YOUR BALANCE

How good is your balance? When we are young, our balance and reaction times are usually good. As we get older, however, things happen that affect our stability such as illness, injury, and medical conditions. Balance is crucial to performing everyday activities and avoiding falls, and it is easy to test our balance at home to get a general idea of how we are doing.

An important thing to remember before testing out your balance on your own is to be honest with yourself and the current condition of your health. It is normal to feel dizzy and off balance if you are ill, under the influence of alcohol or certain medications, or tired. However, if you are experiencing chronic dizziness and balance problems, you should see a doctor to get things checked out. Some warning signs that mean it's time to seek medical evaluation include:

- Periodic episodes of dizziness for no apparent reason.

- Dizziness that lasts for more than two or three days.

- Chronic dizziness that results in the inability to walk or drive safely.

- Dizziness that occurs after a fall or accident.

- Signs of confusion, slurred speech, weakness, or numbness on one side of the body.

Getting prompt diagnosis and a plan for treatment is key to avoiding future problems and increasing chances for a good outcome.

Balance Tests

If you are wondering just how good your balance is, you can do this simple at-home test to get an idea. No equipment is needed.

Balance Test 1: Feet together

- Stand up tall with your feet flat on the floor and ankle bones touching each other.

- Cross your arms in front of your chest.

- Close your eyes.

- Hold this position for as long as you can.

- The standard time to hold this position is 60 seconds.

Balance Test 2: Feet tandem

○   Stand up tall with your feet flat on the floor.

○   Place one foot in front of the other, heel to toe.

○   Close your eyes and hold this position for as long as possible.

○   The standard time to hold this position is 30 seconds.

Balance Test 3: One-legged stand

○   Stand up tall with your feet flat on the floor.

○   Cross your arms in front of your chest.

○   Bend one knee and lift that leg's foot off the floor. Don't allow this leg to touch your other one. Hold this position as long as you can.

○   Now, close your eyes and continue to hold this position for as long as possible.

○   The standard times to hold this position are:

•   Age 60 and younger:

  •   Eyes open: 29 seconds

  •   Eyes closed: 21 seconds

•   Age 61 and older:

  •   Eyes open: 22 seconds

  •   Eyes closed: 10 seconds

Balance Test 4: Alternate one-legged stand

○   Stand up tall with both feet flat on the ground.

○   Put both hands on your hips.

○   Raise one foot and place it against the inside of the calf of your other leg.

○   On your standing leg, raise your heel off the ground so you are standing on the ball of your foot.

○   Hold this position for as long as you can.

○   The standard time for this position is 25 seconds on each leg.

Balance Test 5: Stand and Reach

○   Stand up tall with both feet flat on the ground.

○   Reach forward with both arms out in front of you as far as you can.

○   The standard reach is 10 inches, or 25 centimeters, without losing your balance.

How did you do? If you were not able to hold these positions for their standard times, there is room for improvement in your balance. We will be working on this throughout the remainder of the book.

In this chapter, we covered a lot of information. Understanding how our body regulates our balance and equilibrium gives insight into how and why things can go awry and affect our steadiness. Fall risk factors are real and can be devastating if not addressed, so we also learned how to take preventative measures to ensure we are protected against accidental trips and slips.

What follows in the next few chapters are specific exercises to help our bodies regain and retain good balance. Let's get started!

02 SEATED EXERCISES

"The great thing about getting older is that you don't lose all the other ages you've been.

—Madeleine L'Engle

Those who are not familiar with seated exercising may find it surprising to learn that seated exercises are not only effective, but also a low-impact and safe way to get in some cardio movement, strength training, and flexibility in a low-impact way. Regaining and maintaining your balance can also be accomplished with exercises while in a seated position. If you are recovering from a fall, stroke, or other event that has thrown off your equilibrium, starting with seated exercises is a smart way to start off, as it builds strength and balance while lessening the chance of any further falls. If you are disabled and require a wheelchair, seated exercises may be your only option, depending on the severity of your injuries. But this does not prevent you from completing these exercises and helping you regain and maintain your balance. Sitting requires balance as well and working on your stability will help you to be confident in your sitting posture and abilities to perform other tasks.

In this chapter, we will look at ten of the best seated exercises for balance. For these seated exercises, it is recommended to sit in an armless, straight-backed chair. If you need extra stability, place the chair near a table or low counter that you can place your hand upon if needed.

FORWARD PUNCH

Length of exercise: 20 to 30 seconds

Total time: 5 minutes

Areas worked on: triceps, upper back, lower back, glutes, hamstrings

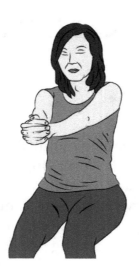 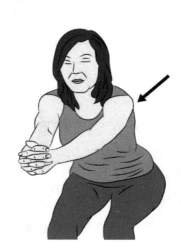

Directions:

1. Sit in the chair with both feet flat on the floor. Raise both arms out straight in front of you with hands clasped together.

2. Slowly lean your upper body forward while keeping your arms in front of you and as if they were reaching for something.

3. Lean as far forward as you can comfortably, hold for five seconds, then slowly return back to the original position. Repeat 10 times.

4. To level up: While leaning forward, reach down towards the floor instead of straight out in front of you. You can also try reaching diagonally.

5. **Take note:** This exercise mimics the everyday activity of reaching for items. Don't lean too far forward if you don't have the core strength. Only lean as far as comfortable for you.

HIP ABDUCTION SIDE KICK

Length of exercise: 2 minutes

Total time: 6 minutes

Areas worked on: abdominals, quadriceps, outside of hip, inner thighs

Seated Exercises
Hip Abduction Side Kick

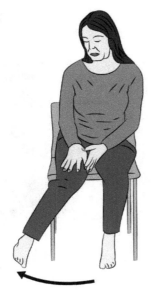 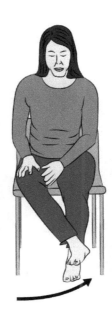

Directions:

1. Sit in the chair with legs about hips-width apart and both feet flat on the floor.

2. Raise up the right leg and right foot off the floor. Kick the right foot out to the side, then swing it back inwards crossing over the left shin. Repeat 20 times.

3. Switch sides using the left leg and foot. Raise the left leg and foot, kicking out to the left and swinging it back in to cross over the right shin. Repeat 20 times.

4. Repeat with both legs two more times each.

5. **Take note:** Be sure to hold on with one or both hands to the sides of the seat or a nearby table for added stability.

HIP EXTERNAL ROTATOR STRETCH

Length of exercise: 2 minutes

Total time: 6 minutes

Areas worked on: glutes, hips, abdominals, lower back

Seated Exercises
Hip External Rotator Stretch

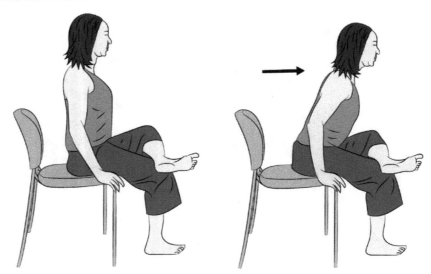

Directions:

1. Sit in the chair with both feet on the floor. Raise the right foot and cross your legs, placing the outside of the right ankle on the left knee.

2. Slowly lean the upper body forward as far as you can. Hands can be on your crossed leg or holding onto the chair. Hold the stretch for 15 to 20 seconds, breathing normally.

3. Return to the starting position. Repeat with the left leg by crossing the left ankle on top of the right knee. Lean forward and hold for 15 to 20 seconds.

4. Repeat two more times on both sides.

5. To level up: Reach for the floor in front of you with both hands.

6. **Take note:** Keeping hips strong and flexible is important for balance and stability. Be sure not to lean too far forward to avoid falling out of the chair.

HIP FLEXION FOLD

Length of exercise: 3 minutes

Total time: 3 minutes

Areas worked on: abdominals, hip flexors, glutes, biceps

Seated Exercises

Hip Flexion Fold

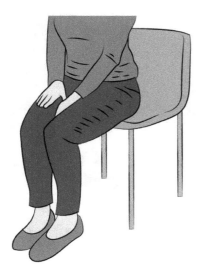 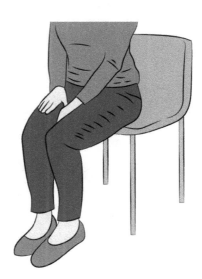

Directions:

1. Sit in the chair with both feet on the floor. Raise the right leg, keeping it bent. Place your hands under your right thigh and draw the leg up as far as you can without bending forward. Hold for three seconds, then lower back down. Repeat 10 times.

2. Switching legs, raise the left leg and place your hands under the left thigh. Draw the leg up and hold for three seconds before lowering back down. Repeat 10 times.

3. **Take note:** Pay attention that your back doesn't start rounding while doing this exercise. Keep sitting up tall and erect with good posture.

ISOMETRIC BACK EXTENSOR HOLD

Length of exercise: 30 seconds

Total time: 5 minutes

Areas worked on: abdominals, upper back, lower back

Seated Exercises
Isometric Back Extensor

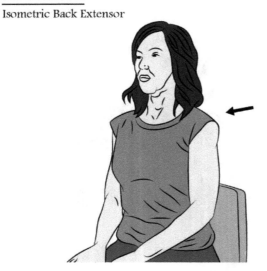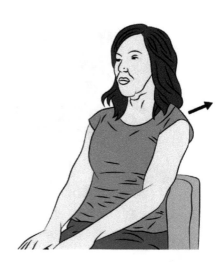

Directions:

1. Sit towards the front edge of the chair with both feet flat on the floor. Slowly lean backwards, slightly rounding your back until you can press your back onto the chair. Hold for five seconds.

2. Slowly return to the original upright position.

3. Repeat 10 times.

4. **Take note:** Be sure not to arch your back when you return to the upright position. For added stability, hold on to the seat with both hands.

LATERAL TRUNK FLEXION

Length of exercise: 1 minute

Total time: 3 minutes

Areas worked on: abdominals, obliques, lower back

Seated Exercises
Lateral Trunk Flexion

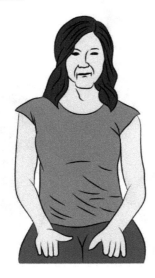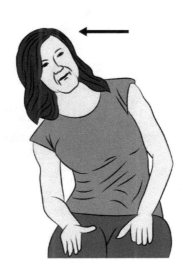

Directions:

1. Sit in the chair with feet on the floor about hips width apart. Sitting upright with hands on the tops of the thighs, slowly tilt to the right, moving your right shoulder towards your right hip as far as you can. Hold for 10 seconds, then return to the original upright position.

2. Switching sides, now slowly tilt to the left, moving your left shoulder towards your left hip as far as you can. Hold for 10 seconds, then return to the original position.

3. Repeat on both sides two more times.

4. **Take note:** Mobility and flexibility in your trunk area helps with stability. Keep your neck and shoulders relaxed and avoid hunching while doing this exercise.

SEATED MARCHING

Length of exercise: 30 seconds

Total time: 1 minute 30 seconds

Areas worked on: abdominals, quadriceps, hamstrings, hip flexors

Seated Exercises
Seated Marching

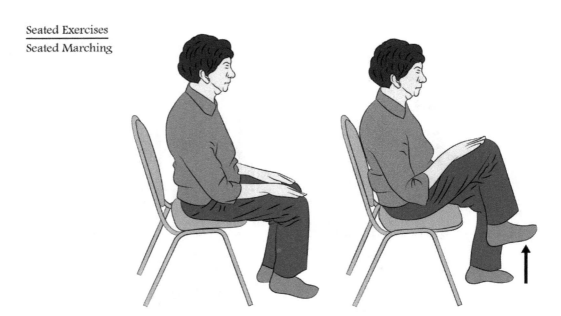

Directions:

1. Sit on the chair close to the front edge, with both feet flat on the floor. Sit up tall without slouching. Hold on to the chair seat with both hands if needed.

2. Pick up the right knee and foot off the floor and lift as high as you can. Be careful not to lean back but remain upright. Put the leg down and switch legs. Lift up the left knee and foot as high as you can. Continue to alternate legs, 'marching' for about 30 seconds.

3. Rest for 30 seconds, then repeat once more.

4. **Take note:** Being able to lift your leg and foot high enough to clear curbs and stairs without losing your balance is an important skill. Don't lean back or let your back start to round as you bring your legs up. Remain sitting up tall and erect.

SIT-TO-STAND

Length of exercise: 30 seconds

Total time: 5 minutes

Areas worked on: abdominals, back, glutes, quadriceps, hamstrings

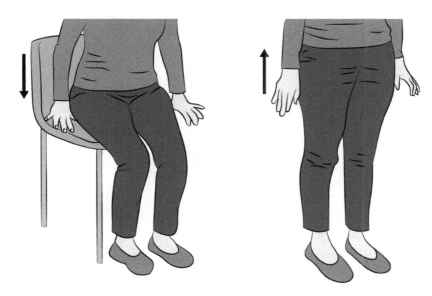

Directions:

1. Sit in a chair with your feet flat on the floor and about hips-width apart. Feet should be slightly behind the knees for leverage.

2. Slowly stand up and remain standing for 10 seconds as you regain balance. Use your hands and arms if needed. Return to a seated position.

3. Repeat 10 times.

4. To level up: Hold a five pound weight between your hands while you do this exercise for added resistance.

5. **Take note:** Going from a sitting to standing position is a daily skill that is needed. Ensure that the chair you use in this exercise is sturdy and will not move as you sit, stand, and return to sit.

TOE RAISES

Length of exercise: 15 seconds

Total time: 2 minutes 30 seconds

Areas worked on: calves, feet

Seated Exercises

Toe Raises

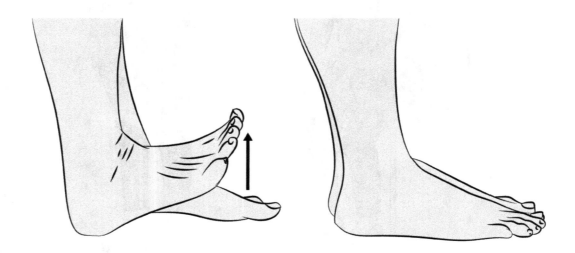

Directions:

1. Sit in a chair with your feet flat on the floor. Place your hands on the tops of your thighs.

2. Slowly raise your toes off the floor. You may notice your upper body wanting to lean back, but stay upright and slightly lean forward if you need to. Hold for 10 seconds, then lower toes back down.

3. Repeat 10 times.

4. To level up: Alternate between raising toes and raising heels.

5. **Take note:** Calf muscle strength is important for ankle stability. If your calf muscles start to burn, take a rest between repetitions.

TRUNK CIRCLES

Length of exercise: 2 minutes

Total time: 6 minutes

Areas worked on: abdominals, obliques, lower back

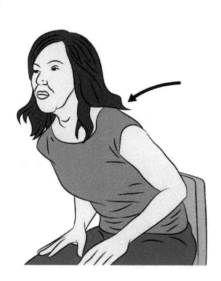 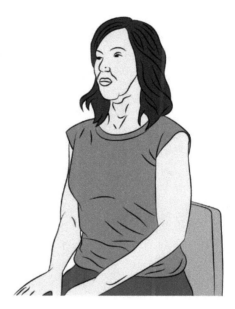

Directions:

1. Sit in a chair with your feet flat on the floor and hips-width apart. Place your hands on top of your thighs.

2. Keep the lower body stationery while you move your shoulders and torso forward, right, back, and left in a clockwise motion. Make 10 big circles. Switch directions and move shoulders and torso forward, left, back, and right in a counter-clockwise motion for 10 circles.

3. Repeat two more times in each direction.

4. To level up: Hold your arms straight out from your sides while doing the exercise.

5. **Take note:** This exercise helps train the body in weight shifts and directional changes. Keep your eyes focused on a stationary object straight in front of you for added balance.

19

03

STANDING EXERCISES

You can't help getting older, but you don't have to get old.

—George Burns

Balance exercises done while standing help improve muscle strength while working on balance. Holding on to the back of a chair, countertop, or railing allows for extra stability while you work on your balance. In this chapter, we look at the 10 best balance exercises to do from a standing position. These standing exercises are dynamic ways to build your balance to accomplish everyday activities and tasks, such as going up and down stairs, turning, stepping in narrow spaces, and reaching for items.

Standing exercises are not only good for strengthening the larger muscles in your legs, like the hamstrings, quadriceps, and calves, it is also key to making the smaller muscles like those in your ankles and feet stronger. Ankle strength and steadiness is an important factor in balance. The loss of ankle strength can lead to challenges in standing, walking, turning around, and even driving.

If you are recovering from an injury or just need extra help, enlist someone to help you as a spotter who will catch you if you lose your balance. As you get stronger and want to make these exercises more challenging, you can adjust your hold. Start off using two hands on a chair or countertop, then level up to using only one hand.

When you find that using one hand is easy, you can then try doing the exercises with only one finger on a chair for balance or maybe even without holding on at all. Go slowly and give yourself time to progress.

3-WAY HIP KICK

Length of exercise: 30 seconds

Total time: 5 minutes

Areas worked on: abdominals, hips

Standing Exercises
3-way hip kick

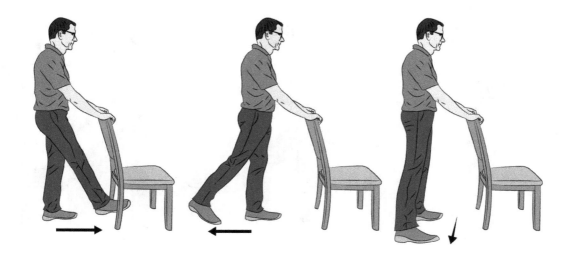

Directions:

1. Stand up tall with your feet about hips-width apart. Place hands on the back of a chair or on a countertop.

2. Extend your right foot and point it out in front of you. Return to the original position. Now extend the right foot out to the right side and then return. Finally, extend the right foot to the back and then return. If the floor was a clock, your right foot would point towards the 12, the 3, and the 6 o'clock positions.

3. Switch legs and now extend the left foot to the front, the left, and the back. Your right foot would point towards the 12, the 9, and the 6 o'clock positions.

4. Repeat 10 times on each leg.

5. **Take note:** Strength in the hip muscles are important for walking, changing direction, and going up and down stairs. Take care not to arch your lower back while completing this exercise.

FOOT TAPS

Length of exercise: 1 minute

Total time: 3 minutes

Areas worked on: abdominals, hip flexor, quadriceps, calves

Standing Exercises

Foot Taps

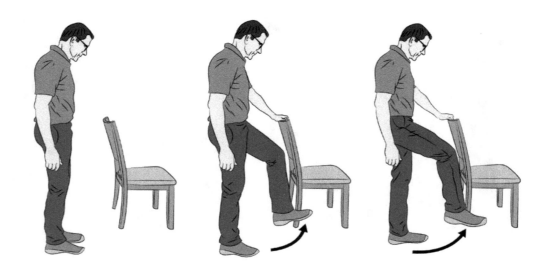

Directions:

1. Place a step stool, thick book, or small cone next to a chair or countertop.

2. Stand up tall with your feet hips-width apart. Hold on to the chair or countertop with both hands.

3. Lift your right foot and tap the step, book, or cone with your toes or ball of the foot. Return your foot to the starting position. Repeat 10 times.

4. Switch legs and lift your left foot and tap the step. Return to the starting position and then repeat 10 times.

5. Repeat each leg two more times.

6. **Take note:** This exercise mimics going up a flight of stairs. Be sure to raise your foot before tapping to avoid stumbling.

HEEL RAISES

Length of exercise: 45 seconds

Total time: 2 minutes

Areas worked on: calves, ankles, feet

Standing Exercises
Heel Raises

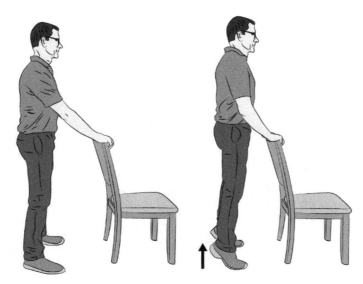

Directions:

1. Stand up tall with your feet hips-width apart. Use both hands to hold on to the back of a chair or countertop.

2. Slowly lift your heels off the ground and feel your weight shift into the front towards your toes. You can use your hands for support, but be sure not to lean your body weight onto them. Lower the heels to the ground. Repeat 10 times.

3. Rest for 15 seconds, then repeat exercise once more.

4. To level up: Use only one hand or one finger on the counter for stability. When comfortable with the exercise, try doing it without the help of any hands.

5. **Take note:** Calf muscles help with ankle stability and overall balance. Be sure you keep good posture while doing this exercise and not lean over onto the counter.

LATERAL STEPPING

Length of exercise: 2 minutes

Total time: 6 minutes

Areas worked on: abdominals, lower back, glutes, quadriceps, hamstrings, calves

Standing Exercises
Lateral Stepping

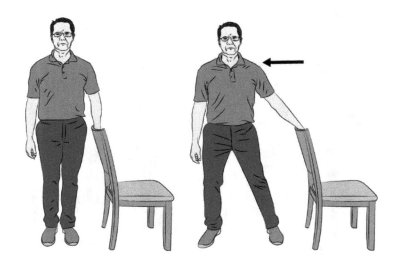

Directions:

1. Stand up tall with your feet together. Hold on to the back of a chair or countertop.

2. Step your right foot out to the side, just past your shoulder, and slightly bend your knee as you put weight on the right foot. Return the foot to the original position. Repeat 10 times.

3. Switch legs and now step your left foot out to the side just past your shoulder. Return the foot to the starting position and repeat 10 times.

4. Repeat exercise two more times on each leg.

5. To level up: Once you are comfortable doing this exercise, try doing it without holding on with your hands.

6. **Take note:** Lateral exercises like this improve coordination in tight spaces. Concentrate on picking up your foot before stepping to avoid tripping. Be sure all loose rugs or other objects are away from the exercise area.

MINI LUNGES

Length of exercise: 2 minutes

Total time: 6 minutes

Areas worked on: abdominals, glutes, quadriceps, hamstrings, calves, ankles

Standing Exercises
Mini Lunges

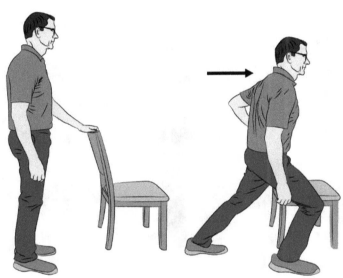

Directions:

1. Stand up tall with feet hips-width apart. Hold on to the back of a chair or countertop.

2. Step your right foot forward and bend your right knee slightly. This is not a deep lunge and should not be painful in any way. Bring your foot back to the starting position. Repeat 10 times.

3. Switch legs and step forward with your left foot, bending the left knee slightly. Bring the foot back to the starting position, then repeat 10 times.

4. Repeat exercise two more times on each leg.

5. To level up: When you are comfortable, use only one finger on the chair for stability.

6. **Take note:** This exercise mimics forward stepping while strengthening the entire leg. Take care to not go too deep in the lunge to avoid straining muscles.

NARROW STANCE REACH

Length of exercise: 2 minutes

Total time: 6 minutes

Areas worked on: shoulders, upper back, lower back, glutes, hamstrings

Standing Exercises
Narrow Stance Reach

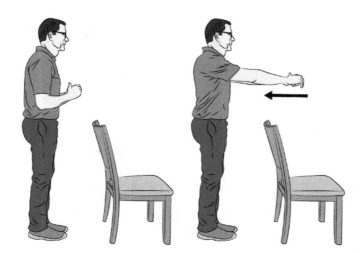

Directions:

1. Stand up tall with feet fairly close together. With your left hand holding on to the back of a chair or countertop, reach forward with the right hand extending as far as it is comfortable. Bring the right hand back to the starting position. Repeat the right hand reaching for 10 times.

2. Switch arms by holding on to the chair with the right hand. Reach forward with the left hand and extend as far as you can. Bring the hand back and repeat the left hand reaching for 10 times.

3. Repeat exercise two more times on each arm.

4. To level up: As you get stronger, you can try reaching with both hands at the same time. You can also reach out to the sides for a directional change.

5. **Take note:** Reaching for items at the back of a cabinet or shelf without losing your balance is an everyday skill. Be sure to keep both feet on the ground to maintain a stable base while reaching.

SINGLE LEG STANCE

Length of exercise: 5 minutes

Total time: 5 minutes

Areas worked on: abdominals, quadriceps, hamstrings, calves, ankles

Standing Exercises

Single Leg Stance

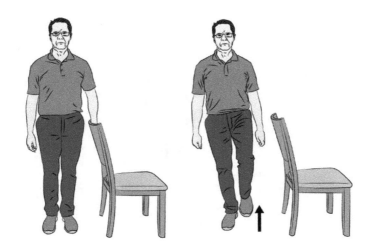

Directions:

1. Stand up tall with feet about hips-width apart. Hold on to the chair or countertop with both hands.

2. Lift the right foot off the floor, continuing to stand tall without leaning too much on the standing leg. Hold for 10 seconds, then lower the right foot back down. Repeat 10 times.

3. Switch legs and lift the left foot off the floor, standing tall, and holding for 10 seconds. Lower the foot and repeat 10 times.

4. **Take note:** We stand on a single leg more than we realize. Everytime you take a step, go up and down stairs, or get into a bathtub, you spend time on one leg. As you progress, do this exercise without holding onto anything with your hands.

SQUATS

Length of exercise: 1 minute

Total time: 2 minutes 15 seconds

Areas worked on: abdominals, lower back, glutes, quadriceps, hamstrings, calves

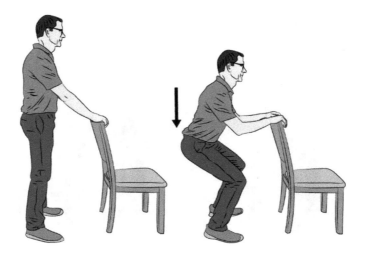

Directions:

1. Stand up tall with your feet hips-width apart. Place your hands on a chair or countertop for stability.

2. Bend both knees and squat, as if you were going to sit down in a chair. Return to a standing position. Repeat 10 times.

3. Rest for 15 seconds, then repeat the exercise 10 more times.

4. To level up: Use only one hand for stability while doing this exercise.

5. **Take note:** Squatting is an essential skill for sitting in a chair or getting into a car. If you are unsure of your ability to come back up from a squat, you can position a sturdy chair behind you that will catch you if you cannot rise from the squat.

STANDING MARCHES

Length of exercise: 1 minute

Total time: 2 minutes

Areas worked on: abdominals, glutes, quadriceps, hamstrings, hip flexors

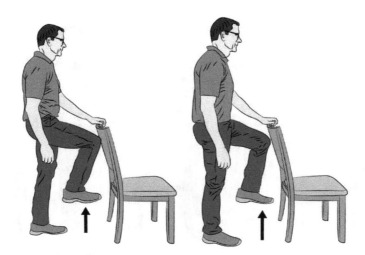

Directions:

1. Stand up tall with your feet hips-width apart. Hold onto a countertop or back of a chair with either your right or left hand.

2. Bend your right leg and raise your right foot as high as you can while remaining upright. Return the right foot to the floor.

3. Bend your left leg and raise your left foot as high as you can, then return it to the floor.

4. Continue 'marching' by lifting one foot and then the other, alternating until you have done it 20 times.

5. Rest if needed, then do the exercise one more time.

6. **Take note:** This exercise helps with single leg balance and the strength of your hips. Be sure to keep good posture and stand up tall while doing this exercise. Avoid rounding your back or hunching forward.

TANDEM STANCE

Length of exercise: 30 seconds

Total time: 5 minutes

Areas worked on: abdominals, lower back, hips

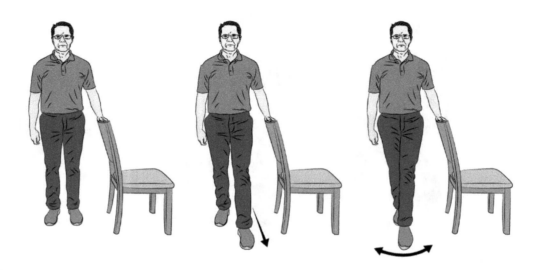

Directions:

1. Stand up tall and hold on to a countertop or the back of a chair with both hands or one hand.

2. Move the right foot and place it directly in front of the left one. Right heel should be in front of the left toes. In this narrow stance, hold the position for 1o seconds.

3. Switch feet by moving the left foot and putting it in front of the right. The left heel should be in front of the right toes. Hold for 10 seconds.

4. Repeat 10 times.

5. **Take note:** Because this exercise causes you to have a narrower base of support, you may feel off balance quickly. Your core muscles will help your stability, so tighten your abs and glutes while doing this exercise.

04 | WALKING EXERCISES

Walking requires balance. Your center of gravity changes each time you take a step, so as you walk, your body is constantly working to maintain equilibrium to keep you upright. Working on your balance as you walk is a good way to incorporate movement into your balance exercises. Training your body in this way helps it to respond to shifts in balance while you are moving and helps to build stability.

It is important to maintain good posture while you are walking. You should be standing straight with your shoulders back and relaxed, with your hands down by your sides. Keep your stomach pulled in and your core tight to prevent any leaning forward or backwards, which can put a strain on your back. It's also good to keep your chin parallel to the ground and your gaze looking ahead of you to reduce any pressure on your neck as well as being able to spot what's ahead on your path. Regularly check your posture at intervals during your walk and make adjustments in it to build good posture habits. Over time, your body will gravitate towards keeping a good alignment and posture.

In this chapter, we look at the ten easy ways to incorporate balance exercises while walking across a room. You can also do these while on your daily walks in your neighborhood or on a treadmill. If you are recovering from injury or have trouble walking, be sure to have a companion that can walk with you and assist you if needed.

BACKWARD WALKING

Length of exercise: 30 seconds

Total time: 3 minutes

Areas worked on: abdominals, glutes, hips, quadriceps, hamstrings, calves, ankles

Walking Exercises
Backward Walk

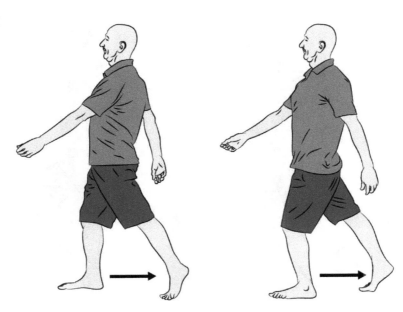

Directions:

1. This exercise is best done with a partner that can alert you to any tripping hazards. Be sure to walk on a flat, level area. If you are on a sidewalk, make sure you are away from traffic and other pedestrians. This can also be done on a treadmill.

2. To start, walk forward 10 steps. Turn around and continue to walk in the same direction but facing backwards. Walk slowly for 10 steps. Turn around again and continue to walk 10 steps forward.

3. Repeat for 2 minutes, alternating between walking 10 steps facing forward and 10 steps facing backward all while walking in one direction.

4. To level up: Once you are comfortable walking backwards, walk for 20 steps instead of 10 steps.

5. **Take note:** This exercise helps your core muscles respond to directional changes as well as working your leg muscles in different ways. Take care not to walk too quickly when walking backwards to avoid falling.

BALANCE WALKING

Length of exercise: 1 minute 30 seconds

Total time: 3 minutes

Areas worked on: shoulders, abdominals, hip flexors, glutes, hamstrings, ankles

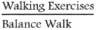

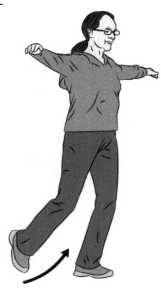
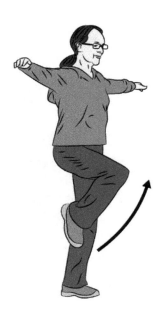

Directions:

1. Standing up tall, bring your arms up and out straight from the sides of your body to about shoulder height.

2. Take one step forward with your right foot and as you bring your left foot from behind you to take the next step, bend your left knee and lift your left foot up. Pause for 1 second before following through with the rest of the step forward with your left foot.

3. Do the same thing now with your right foot. As you bring your right leg forward for the next step, bend your right knee and lift the right foot, holding it up for 1 second before completing the step. Repeat for 20 steps.

4. Rest for a few seconds, then repeat exercise once more.

5. **Take note:** This exercise is similar to the standing marches but with forward movement. The ankle muscles are being strengthened as they help your body stabilize. If you need support, have a partner hold one of your hands.

BALL TOSS

Length of exercise: 30 seconds

Total time: 1 minute 30 seconds

Areas worked on: hands, forearms, glutes, hip flexors, hamstrings, calves

Walking Exercises
Ball Toss

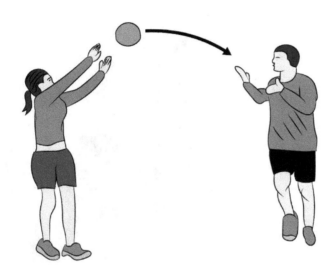

Directions:

1. Bring a small squishy ball with you on your walk. As you walk forward, squish the ball in your right hand as you walk 10 steps forward.

2. Toss the ball to your left hand and squish the ball in your left hand as you continue walking for another 10 steps.

3. Repeat two more times in each hand.

4. **Take note:** By having to multitask, your body will adjust its balance and coordination. Be sure you keep your eyes focused on where you are walking to avoid tripping.

CURB WALKING

Length of exercise: 30 seconds

Total time: 30 seconds

Areas worked on: abdominals, hips, glutes, inner thighs, hamstrings, calves

Walking Exercises
Curb Walking

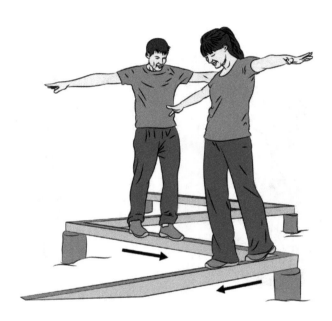

Directions:

1. Try walking in a straight line on a slightly raised surface like a two-by-four length of wood or a curb. If you are outside, be sure that you are walking somewhere away from traffic and with a friend. You can place your hand on their shoulder for support or hold their arm.

2. If you are unsure about walking on something as tall as a curb, try walking in a straight line, heel-to-toe, on a flat path.

3. **Take note:** This exercise requires a narrower stance, which gives you a smaller base of stability. Walk slow and heel-to-toe to avoid falling off the curb.

DYNAMIC WALKING

Length of exercise: 30 seconds

Total time: 5 minutes

Areas worked on: neck, abdominals, hip flexors, glutes, hamstrings, calves

Walking Exercises
Dynamic Walking

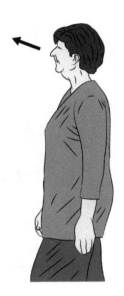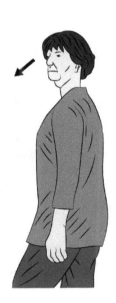

Directions:

1. Do this first in your living room or backyard until you get used to it. Starting at one end of your room or yard, walk slowly towards the opposite side.

2. While continuing to walk straight, slowly turn your head to the right and then to the left while walking. Continue turning your head to the right and left slowly until you reach the other side of the room.

3. Repeat 10 times.

4. To level up: As you get more confident, you can incorporate this into your walks outside at the park or in your neighborhood.

5. **Take note:** This exercise requires a shift in your focus each time you turn your head. Be sure to turn your head slowly to avoid dizziness. If you feel dizzy at any time, stop.

GRAPEVINE

Length of exercise: 1 minutes

Total time: 5 minutes

Areas worked on: abdominals, hips, inner thighs, quadriceps, calves

Walking Exercises

Grapevine

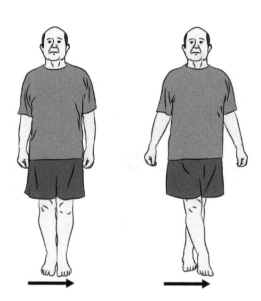

Directions:

1. You can hold onto a countertop as you do this exercise or have a partner hold on to your hands if you feel unsteady.

2. Start by standing up tall with your feet together. Cross your right foot over your left and step down. Uncross by bringing your left foot back and place it next to your right so both feet are together normally. Continue crossing your right foot over your left for 10 steps or until you reach the other end of the countertop.

3. Go back in the other direction by now crossing your left foot behind your right and stepping to the right. Uncross by bringing your right foot up and placing it next to your left. Continue crossing your left foot behind as you travel to the right for 10 steps or reach the end of the counter.

4. Repeat five times.

5. To level up: If you get very comfortable with this exercise, you can make it more challenging by alternating crossing in front and crossing behind every other step.

6. **Take note:** At first you may find yourself looking down at your feet, but remember to look up and see where you are going. Try to keep your head up.

40

HEEL-TO-TOE

Length of exercise: 30 seconds

Total time: 2 minutes 30 seconds

Areas worked on: abdominals, hips, inner thighs, quadriceps, hamstrings, calves

Walking Exercises
Heel-to-Toe

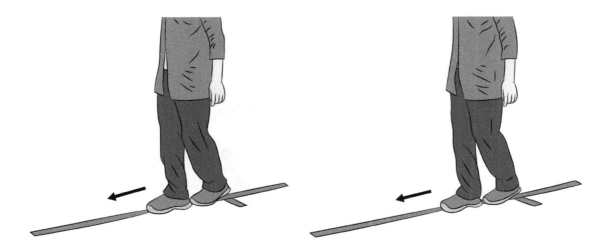

Directions:

1. You can hold onto a countertop as you do this exercise or have a partner hold on to your hands if you feel unsteady.

2. Stand up tall and put your right foot directly in front of your left. Walk heel-to-toe as if you were walking on a tightrope. Continue walking heel-to-toe for 15 steps or until you reach the other end of the counter or opposite side of the room.

3. Repeat five times.

4. To level up: To make this more challenging, you can place masking tape or blue painters tape in a straight line on your floor. Practice walking on the line, without holding onto anything.

5. **Take note:** This exercise requires a narrower stance and will challenge your balance because of a smaller base of support. You can raise your arms away from your sides to help with stability if you are not holding onto anything.

SIDE STEPS

Length of exercise: 45 seconds

Total time: 4 minutes

Areas worked on: abdominals, hip abductors, quadriceps, glutes, calves

Walking Exercises
Side Steps

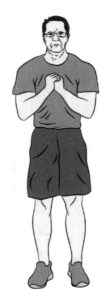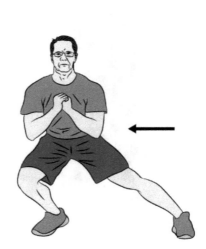

Directions:

1. Practice this first in your living room or backyard until you are confident in your ability. Standing up tall, step to the right with your right foot and bring your left foot to meet your right. Continue sidestepping to the right 10 times.

2. Change direction and now step to the left with your left foot. Bring your right foot to meet your left and continue sidestepping to the left 10 times.

3. Repeat five times.

4. To level up: Once you are self-assured in this move, you can practice this on your walks outside. Turn sideways while walking and side step for 10 steps in one direction before switching to the other side. Remember to always keep your head facing the direction you are moving.

5. **Take note:** Sidestepping is an everyday skill that you use at home, in stores, and anywhere there are people around. Avoid looking down at your feet. Instead look straight ahead or in the direction you are moving.

WALK ON HEELS AND TOES

Length of exercise: 30 seconds

Total time: 1 minute 30 seconds

Areas worked on: abdominals, hip flexors, calves

Walking Exercises
Heel-to-Toe

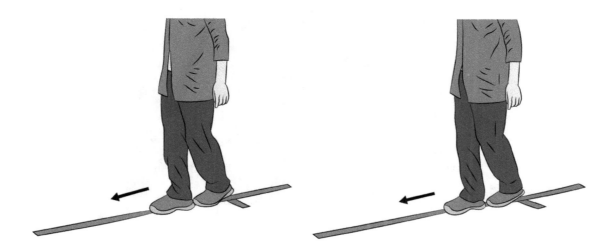

Directions:

1. Be sure to warm up your legs and feet by walking normally for five minutes before starting this exercise. You can hold onto a countertop or enlist the help of a friend if you need added support.

2. Walk slowly forward on your heels with your toes lifted off the ground. Walk for 10 steps.

3. Walk forward normally for 10 steps.

4. Now, slowly walk on your toes with your heels lifted off the ground. Walk for 10 steps.

5. Repeat two times.

6. **Take note:** If your calves or feet are starting to cramp, take a break, and do only half the steps. Increase the amount of steps only when you are comfortable.

ZIGZAG WALKING

Length of exercise: 1 minute

Total time: 5 minutes

Areas worked on: abdominals, hips, quadriceps, hamstrings, calves

Walking Exercises
Zigzag Walk

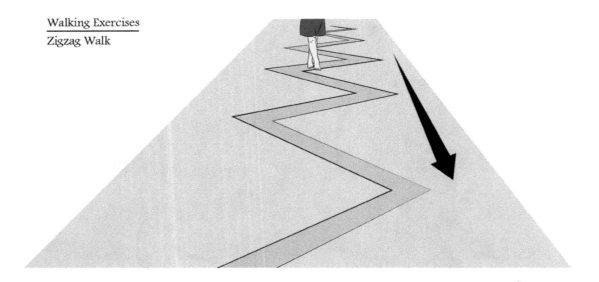

Directions:

1. This exercise requires directional shifts to increase your balance while walking. You can set up two cones six feet apart and walk in a figure eight pattern around the cones. Repeat five times.

2. Alternatively, you can walk in a zigzag pattern on a path or sidewalk. Walk forward at an angle towards the right side of the path, then walk forward towards the left side of the path. Zigzag back and forth across the path several times.

3. **Take note:** Because walking in a serpentine pattern means a change in directions, your balance will be challenged. Keep your core muscles engaged as you walk.

05 | CORE EXERCISES

Aging has a wonderful beauty and we should have respect for that.

—Eartha Kitt

Our core is the area from the lower ribs all the way down the trunk of the body to the buttocks. The core muscles are important for balance and stabilization in our bodies. These muscles include the muscles in the stomach and belly area, the obliques on the side of the body, and the back muscles. They are important in helping us complete everyday tasks such as getting out of bed, sitting, standing, and bending over. Providing stability to the back, arms, and legs, the core muscles need regular exercise to remain strong. When these muscles are exercised, they also help support a healthy back and minimize back pain.

There was a time when core exercises consisted mainly of sit-ups and crunches. These used to be the gold standard to not only getting a trim midsection but also a strong core. But as we get older, these exercises can cause problems with our aging necks and backs. Pulling on your neck and pushing your spine against a hard surface, even if it is lightly padded, is hard on your entire back. Degenerative disc disease, back problems, and arthritis can also make sit-ups and crunches painful and difficult. Additionally, those exercises only work a few stomach muscles and not the rest of the core. Sit-ups and crunches mainly target the hip flexors, which are the muscles that run along the lower back to the thighs. Overworking the hip flexors can cause them to become overly strong or too tight, resulting in lower back pain and discomfort.

In this chapter, we will learn ten of the best exercises to strengthen your core and how to exercise a variety of core muscles. When we train the entire set of core muscles, instead of just a few muscles in isolation, we are having those muscles work together like they do in our everyday movements.

BRIDGE

Length of exercise: 30 seconds

Total time: 5 minutes

Areas worked on: lower back, glutes, hamstrings, calves

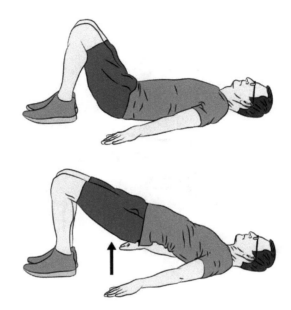

Core Exercises
Bridge

Directions:

1. Lie on your back facing up on the floor or a padded mat. Bend your knees and keep your feet flat on the floor about hips-width apart. Arms should be on the floor by your sides.

2. Tighten up your buttocks. Lift your hips off the floor so that your lower back and mid back are also off the floor. Your shoulders, hips, and knees should form a straight line. Hold for 10 seconds, then gently lower to the floor.

3. Repeat 10 times.

4. **Take note:** The closer your feet are to your glutes, the harder it will be to lift your hips off the floor, so adjust the distance accordingly. Remember to lower back down to the floor with control.

FOREARM PLANK

Length of exercise: 30 seconds

Total time: 2 minutes 30 seconds

Areas worked on: shoulders, upper back, abdominals

Core Exercises
Forearm Plank

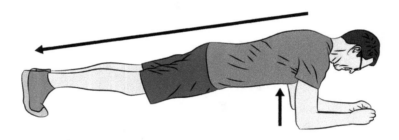

Directions:

1. Facing the ground or a mat on the floor, lie face down with your forearms on the ground. Be sure that your elbows are directly under your shoulders and that your back is not arching.

2. Tighten your core and press into your forearms and toes to lift your body off the floor. Press your belly button in towards your spine and squeeze your buttocks to help stabilize your body and keep it in a straight line. Hold for 20 seconds. Slowly lower to the floor.

3. Repeat five times.

4. To level up: Support your body on your hands instead of your forearms. Hands should be flat on the floor directly under the shoulders.

5. **Take note:** Do not allow your hips to sag, causing a sway in the lower back. Your body should be in a straight diagonal line from your shoulders to feet.

MODIFIED PLANK

Length of exercise: 30 seconds

Total time: 2 minutes 30 seconds

Areas worked on: shoulders, upper back, abdominals

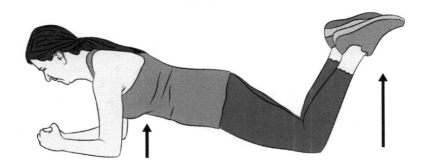

Directions:

1. Start with your hands and knees on the floor and your gaze facing down.

2. Lower your forearms down to the floor and support your upper body on them. Your knees, hips, and shoulders should form a straight line like in a regular plank. Hold the position for 30 seconds. Slowly lower to the ground.

3. Repeat five times.

4. **Take note:** This is the modified version of the forearm plank for those who are still building core strength. If you have any knee issues, you may want to put a folded towel or other padding under your knees.

OPPOSITE ARM AND LEG RAISE

Length of exercise: 1 minute

Total time: 3 minutes

Areas worked on: shoulders, upper back, lower back, glutes, hamstrings

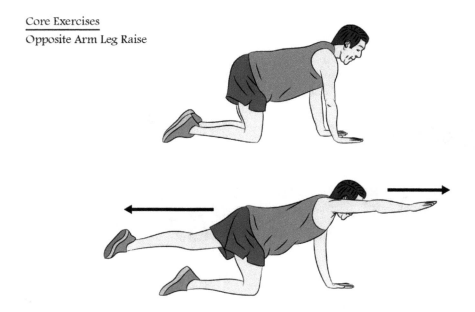

Core Exercises
Opposite Arm Leg Raise

Directions:
1. Start with your hands and knees on the floor and your gaze facing down. Keep your neck neutral and in line with your spine.

2. Straighten your right leg and extend your right foot behind you, toes pointing down to the ground. Try to bring your leg up so it is parallel to the floor. If you can, raise the opposite arm, your left arm, and extend it out in front of you while still looking down. Hold the position for 10 seconds, then slowly lower your arm and leg back down to the ground. Repeat five times.

3. Switch sides by now straightening your left leg and foot out behind you. Raise your right arm and extend it out in front of you. Hold the position for 10 seconds, then slowly lower back to the ground. Repeat on this side five times.

4. Repeat the exercise on both sides twice more.

5. **Take note:** If keeping your arm up is too challenging, you can hold on to something sturdy in front of you, like a chair or table leg to help with balance.

SEATED FORWARD ROLL UP

Length of exercise: 30 seconds

Total time: 5 minutes

Areas worked on: abdominals

Core Exercises

Seated Forward Roll-Ups

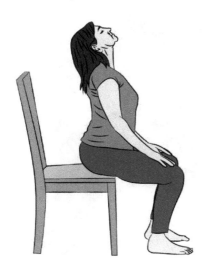 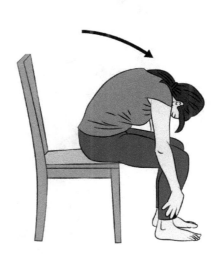

Directions:

1. Sit up tall in a chair towards the front edge of the seat. Extend your legs straight out in front of you with your feet on the floor and flexed toward you.

2. Extend your arms out in front of you and slowly lower your chin towards your chest. Roll your back and chest forward as you reach your hands towards your feet. Engage your abdominal muscles to hold you steady.

3. Once you have reached your hands as far as you can, slowly roll back up to the starting position.

4. Repeat 10 times.

5. **Take note:** Remember to go slowly and not use momentum in this exercise.

SEATED HALF ROLL-BACKS

Length of exercise: 30 seconds

Total time: 5 minutes

Areas worked on: abdominals, upper back, lower back

Core Exercises

Seated Half Roll Backs

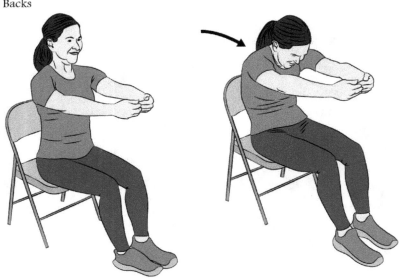

Directions:

1. Sit up tall in a chair towards the front edge of the seat. Keep your knees bent and feet flat on the floor.

2. Lift your arms out in front of you so they form a circle with your fingertips touching. Round your back and tighten your abdominal muscles as you bring your chin to your chest. Hold the position for 10 seconds, then slowly roll up and return to the starting position.

3. Repeat 10 times.

4. **Take note:** Be sure to start with an upright posture before rounding and return to the same upright position. Don't slouch or lean back into the chair.

SEATED LEG LIFTS

Length of exercise: 30 seconds

Total time: 5 minutes

Areas worked on: abdominals, hip flexors, quadriceps

Core Exercises
Seated Leg Lift

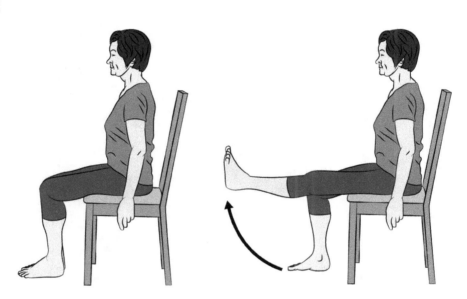

Directions:

1. Sit up tall in a chair with your knees bent and feet flat on the floor. Hands can be on the tops of your thighs or holding on the sides of the seat.

2. Slowly straighten the right leg and lift the right foot off the floor. Try to bring the right leg as high as you can but don't let your back start to round. Keep your back upright and straight. Hold your leg up for five seconds, then slowly lower to the starting position.

3. Switch legs by straightening your left leg and lifting the left foot off the floor. Bring it up as high as you can and hold for five seconds. Slowly lower to the starting position.

4. Repeat each leg 10 times.

5. To level up: Once you are stronger, try doing the exercise with your arms straight out in front of you.

6. **Take note:** Don't let your back become round or collapse as you lift your leg.

SEATED LEG TAPS

Length of exercise: 30 seconds

Total time: 5 minutes

Areas worked on: abdominals, hip flexors, quadriceps

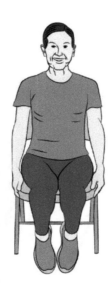 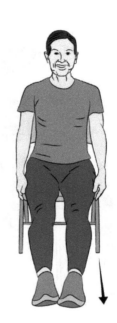

Directions:

1. Sit up tall in a chair with your knees bent and feet flat on the floor. Place your hands on the sides of the seat for support.

2. Tighten your abdominal muscles and straighten both legs out in front of you, lifting both feet off the floor. Try to bring the legs parallel to the floor. Slowly lower your right foot and tap the floor. Bring it back up. Slowly lower your left foot and tap the floor. Bring it back up.

3. Continue alternating tapping the right foot and then the left.

4. Repeat 10 times.

5. To level up: To make it more challenging, raise and lower both feet at the same time.

6. **Take note:** If you need to take a break, lower both feet to the floor for a quick rest before repeating the exercise.

SEATED SIDE BENDS

Length of exercise: 1 minute

Total time: 5 minutes

Areas worked on: abdominals, obliques

Core Exercises

Seated Side Bends

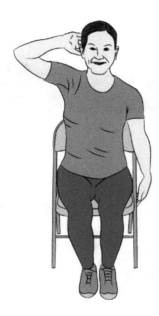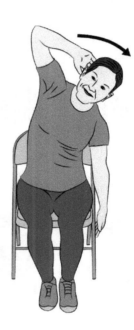

Directions:

1. Sit up tall in a chair with your knees bent and feet flat on the floor. Arms should be hanging at your sides.

2. Bend and raise your right arm, placing your right hand gently on the side of your head while looking straight ahead. Bend at the waist and lean your upper body to the left. Extend your left hand down towards the floor as far as you can as you continue looking straight ahead. Slowly come back up to the starting position. Repeat 10 times.

3. Switch sides and raise your left arm, placing your left hand on the side of your head. Extend your right hand down towards the floor as you bend at the waist and lean to the right. Remember to keep looking straight ahead. Come back up to the starting position. Repeat 1o times.

4. Rest, then repeat the exercise one more time on both sides.

5. To level up: Straighten your bent arm above your head as you lean your body to the side.

6. **Take note:** Pay attention to your neck and shoulders. Don't hunch up. Keep your shoulders down and away from your ears.

SUPERMAN

Length of exercise: 30 seconds

Total time: 5 minutes

Areas worked on: abdominals, upper back, lower back, hip flexors, glutes

Core Exercises

Superman

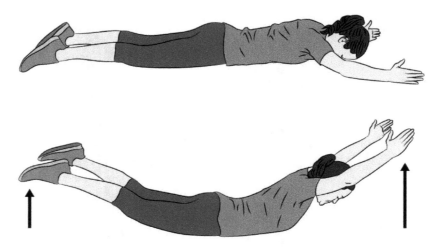

Directions:

1. Lie on the floor or a padded mat, facing down. Extend your arms out straight over your head and legs out straight out behind you. Your body should form a straight line.

2. Tighten the abdominal muscles as you lift your hands and feet off the floor. Keep your neck neutral and gaze looking at the floor. Hold the lifted position for 10 seconds, then slowly lower back down to the ground.

3. Repeat 10 times.

4. **Take note:** To avoid straining your neck, keep your gaze down and look at the floor.

06 VESTIBULAR EXERCISES

Nothing matters more than your health. Healthy living is priceless. What millionaire wouldn't pay dearly for an extra 10 or 20 years of healthy aging?

—Peter Diamandis

Our brains interpret the information that it receives from our eyes, ears, and other senses. If there is an injury or something happens to disrupt the way the brain receives this input, that can result in equilibrium and balance problems. The resulting dizziness can make day to day activities like walking, turning, and driving more challenging. Retraining the brain with exercises that induce dizziness in a controlled manner and the means to overcome it helps build up strength and tolerance in the vestibular system. If you are having dizziness, it is important to first visit your doctor to get it checked out and identify the root cause of it.

Vestibular exercises can help us regain any balance that has been lost. These exercises train the eyes and brain to interpret the information being received and, initially, they may cause some dizziness. To avoid any injury or falls, do these exercises while seated.

EYES SIDE-TO-SIDE

Length of exercise: 30 seconds

Total time: 1 minute

Areas worked on: ocular muscles

Vestibular Exercises
Eyes Side To Side

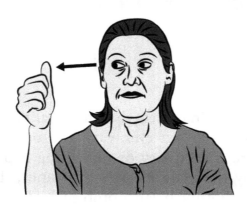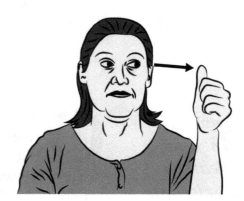

Directions:

1. Sit up tall in a chair with your knees bent and feet flat on the floor. Hold on to the seat or to a tabletop with one hand.

2. Raise the other arm out in front of you. Focus your eyes on your index finger. Move your finger to the right of you and to the left and follow your finger, moving only your eyes. Keep your head still while your eyes move. Move your finger back and forth 10 to 20 times.

3. Rest for a few seconds and repeat once more.

4. **Take note:** If you feel yourself getting dizzy, stop and close your eyes for a moment.

EYES UP AND DOWN

Length of exercise: 30 seconds

Total time: 1 minute

Areas worked on: ocular muscles

Vestibular Exercises
Eyes Up And Down

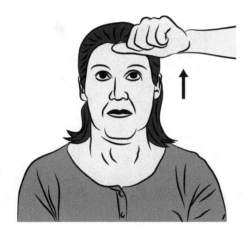 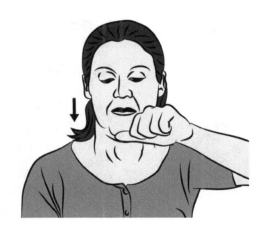

Directions:

1. Sit up tall in a chair with your knees bent and feet flat on the floor. Hold on to the seat or to a tabletop with one hand.

2. Raise the other arm out in front of you. Focus your eyes on your index finger. Move your finger up towards the ceiling then down towards the floor. Keeping your head still, follow your finger with only your eyes. Move your finger up and down 10 to 20 times.

3. **Take note:** Keep your head still and level, with your chin parallel to the floor. Only your eyes should be moving.

GAZE STABILIZATION SITTING

Length of exercise: 30 seconds

Total time: 1 minute

Areas worked on: ocular muscles, neck

Vestibular Exercises
Gaze Stabilization Sitting

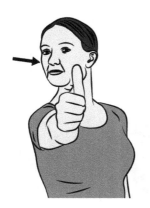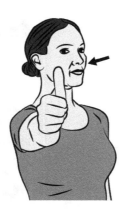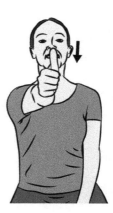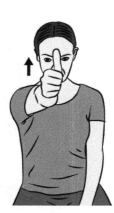

Directions:

1. Sit up tall in a chair with your knees bent and feet flat on the floor. Hold on to the seat or to a tabletop with one or both hands.

2. Focus your eyes on an object or picture three to ten feet away from you. Preferably this object or picture will have a blank, not patterned wall behind it. While keeping your eyes focused on the object, turn your head to the right, then to the left. Keep moving your head from side to side while remaining focused on the object. Turn side to side 20 to 30 times.

3. **Take note:** Take care to hold on to the seat or tabletop to avoid potential falling.

GAZE STABILIZATION STANDING

Length of exercise: 30 seconds

Total time: 1 minute

Areas worked on: ocular muscles, neck

Vestibular Exercises

Gaze Stabilization Standing

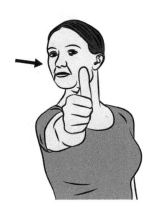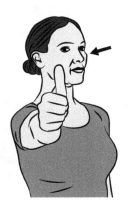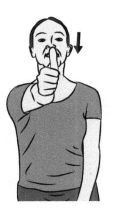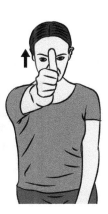

Directions:

1. Stand up tall with both hands on the back of a chair or on a countertop.

2. Focus your eyes on an object or picture three to ten feet away from you. Preferably this object or picture will have a blank, not patterned wall behind it. While keeping your eyes focused on the object, move your head up, then down. Keep moving your head up and down while remaining focused on the object. Move your head up and down 20 to 30 times.

3. **Take note:** To avoid falling, ensure that the chair you are holding on to is sturdy.

HEAD AND EYES OPPOSITE DIRECTION

Length of exercise: 30 seconds

Total time: 1 minute

Areas worked on: ocular muscles, neck

Vestibular Exercises
Head And Eyes Opposite Direction

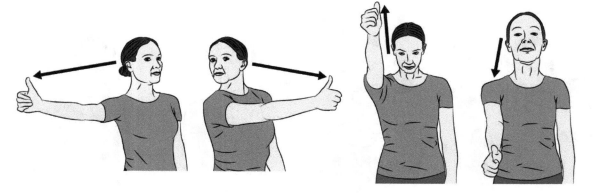

Directions:

1. Sit up tall in a chair with your knees bent and feet flat on the floor. Hold on to the seat or to a tabletop with one hand.

2. In the other hand, hold a pencil or other small object out in front of you. While keeping your eyes focused on the pencil, move the pencil to the right as you move your head to the left. Reverse the motion by moving the pencil to the left as you move your head to the right and keep focusing on the pencil with your eyes. Repeat 20 times.

3. Rest and repeat exercise once more.

4. To level up: As you get better at this exercise, you can do it standing up.

5. **Take note:** Do this exercise slowly and avoid hunching up your shoulders.

HEAD AND EYES SAME DIRECTION

Length of exercise: 30 seconds

Total time: 1 minute

Areas worked on: ocular muscles, neck

Vestibular Exercises
Head And Eyes Same Direction

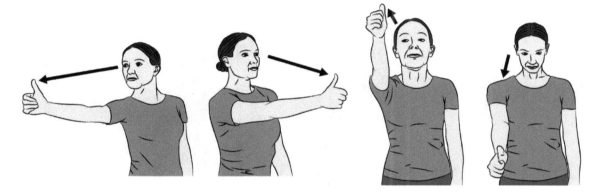

Directions:

1. Sit up tall in a chair with your knees bent and feet flat on the floor. Hold on to the seat or to a tabletop with one hand.

2. In the other hand, hold a pencil or other small object out in front of you. While keeping your eyes focused on the pencil, move it to the right and allow your head and eyes to follow it. Reverse the motion and move the pencil to the left, moving your head and eyes along with it.

3. You can change direction and move the object up and down, allowing your head and eyes to follow. Repeat 20 times.

4. Rest and repeat once more.

5. To level up: Once you are comfortable with the exercise, try doing it standing up.

6. **Take note:** Keep your shoulders and upper body fairly stationary. Avoid leaning over as you move the object up and down.

HEAD BEND

Length of exercise: 30 seconds

Total time: 2 minutes

Areas worked on: ocular muscles, neck

Vestibular Exercises
Head Bend

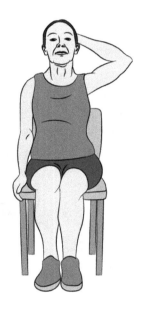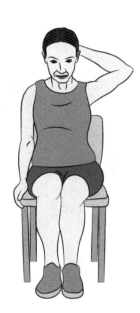

Directions:

1. Sit up tall in a chair with your knees bent and feet flat on the floor. Hold on to the seat or to a tabletop with one or both hands.

2. Bend your neck and head to look down at the floor, then bring them up to look at the ceiling. Let your eyes lead your head as you continue to look down and then up 10 times.

3. Rest and repeat two times.

4. To level up: Do the exercise while standing.

5. **Take note:** Keep your posture tall and upright while doing the exercise. Don't lean forward or backwards.

HEAD TURN

Length of exercise: 30 seconds

Total time: 2 minutes

Areas worked on: ocular muscles, neck

Vestibular Exercises
Head Turn

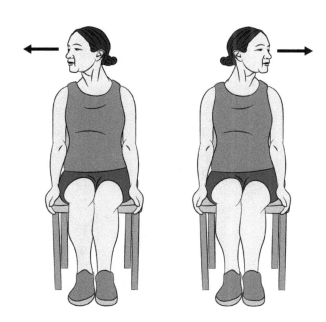

Directions:

1. Sit up tall in a chair with your knees bent and feet flat on the floor. Hold on to the seat or to a tabletop with one or both hands.

2. Turn your neck and head to the right as you look to the right with your eyes. Then turn your neck and head to the left as you look left. Let your eyes lead your head as you continue to look right and left, as if you were watching a tennis match, for 10 times.

3. Rest and repeat two times.

4. To level up: Stand up tall and hold on to a chair while doing the exercise.

5. **Take note:** Only turn your eyes and your head, not your whole body.

SHOULDER TURNS

Length of exercise: 1 minute

Total time: 3 minutes

Areas worked on: abdominals, obliques, upper back, lower back

Vestibular Exercises
Shoulder Turn

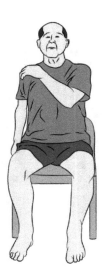 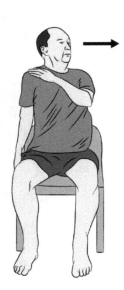

Directions:

1. Sit up tall in a chair with your knees bent and feet flat on the floor. Hold on to the seat with one or both hands.

2. Rotate your head and upper body as you turn to the right, then to the left, keeping your eyes open. Repeat 20 times.

3. Do the exercise again, but this time with your eyes closed as you turn to the right and left. Repeat 20 times.

4. Rest and repeat two more times.

5. To level up: If you are comfortable, do this exercise while standing and holding onto a chair or countertop.

6. **Take note:** It may be helpful to have a partner to help you while you do this with your eyes closed to ensure you don't fall.

SMOOTH PURSUITS

Length of exercise: 30 seconds

Total time: 1 minute 30 seconds

Areas worked on: ocular muscles

Vestibular Exercises
Smooth Pursuits

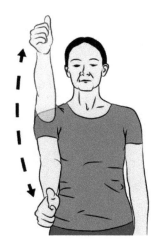 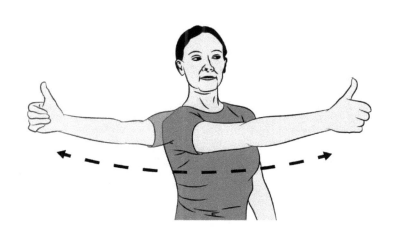

Directions:

1. Sit up tall in a chair with your knees bent and feet flat on the floor. Hold on to the seat or to a tabletop with one hand.

2. Hold a pencil or small object in the other hand. Keeping your head still, move the pencil in a diagonal fashion while your eyes follow the moving object. Move the object from the lower left to upper right and vice versa, or in a zigzag pattern. Repeat 20 times.

3. Rest and repeat two times.

4. Take note: Remember to keep your head still and move your eyes only.

07 EXERCISE ROUTINES

We have looked at 50 exercises that can help strengthen your body and brain to regain and maintain balance. That number of exercises may seem overwhelming to you, especially if you don't have a plan to incorporate them into your daily schedule. It is important to have a plan to utilize the information here so that each day, you can just "plug and play" your exercise routine.

Some options for exercise routines include:

- **One a day.** Methodically working through each exercise on your own schedule. Do one exercise a day until you work through all 50 exercises.

- **Chapter focused.** Another alternative is to work through the exercises chapter-by-chapter. For instance, if you did one move a day from the chapter on seated exercises, you would complete them all in ten days. If you did two moves a day, you would complete the chapter in five days.

- **Routines.** Finally, you can follow the carefully crafted routines that are presented in this chapter. There is a month's worth of exercise plans. The routines are weekly, five days a week. The schedules include a week focused on core moves, a week concentrating on leg strength, a week devoted to brain training, and, finally, a week of walking and movement.

CORE FOCUS WEEK

The concentration of this weekly routine is core strength and foundational seated exercises. As we learned in an earlier chapter, the core muscles include the abdominal, back, and glute muscles. These muscles provide needed stabilization for your body, arms, and legs to move about and function. Strong core muscles also help alleviate back pain while building balance.

Day 1

- Bridge (Ch. 5)
- Modified Plank (Ch. 5)
- Superman (Ch. 5)
- Hip External Rotator Stretch (Ch. 2)

Day 2

- Seated Forward Roll Up (Ch. 5)
- Seated Side Bend (Ch. 5)
- Seated Marching (Ch. 2)
- Isometric Back Extensor (Ch. 2)

Day 3

- Forearm Plank (Ch. 5)
- Opposite Arm and Leg Raise (Ch. 5)
- Lateral Trunk Flexion (Ch. 2)
- Forward Punch (Ch. 2)

Day 4

- Seated Half Roll-Backs (Ch. 5)
- Seated Leg Lifts (Ch. 5)
- Seated Leg Taps (Ch. 5)

    ○   Hip Abduction Side Kicks (Ch. 2)

Day 5

    ○   Hip Flexion (Ch. 2)

    ○   Toe Raises (Ch. 2)

    ○   Sit-to-Stand (Ch. 2)

    ○   Trunk Circles (Ch. 2)

LEG STRENGTH WEEK

The objective of this week's exercises is to build strength and balance in the lower half of the body, particularly the legs. Falls, strokes, and accidents can result in one leg being weaker than the other, causing imbalances over time. The exercises this week will concentrate on strengthening both legs and the lower body while maintaining equilibrium.

Day 1

    ○   Seated Marching (Ch. 2)

    ○   Hip External Rotator Stretch (Ch. 2)

    ○   Single Leg Stance (Ch. 3)

    ○   Foot Taps (Ch. 3)

Day 2

    ○   Hip Flexion Fold (Ch. 2)

    ○   Sit-to-Stand (Ch. 2)

    ○   Standing Marches (Ch. 3)

    ○   Squats (Ch. 3)

Day 3

    ○   Hip Abduction Side Kicks (Ch. 2)

    ○   Seated Leg Lifts (Ch. 5)

    ○   3-Way Hip Kicks (Ch. 3)

- o   Mini Lunges (Ch.3)

Day 4
- o   Seated Leg Taps (Ch. 5)
- o   Narrow Stance Reach (Ch. 3)
- o   Lateral Stepping (Ch. 3)
- o   Heel Raises (Ch. 3)

Day 5
- o   Bridge (Ch. 5)
- o   Opposite Arm and Leg Raise (Ch. 5)
- o   Tandem Stance (Ch. 3)
- o   Walk on Tiptoes (Ch. 4)

BRAIN TRAINING WEEK

This week's schedule is focused on the brain and head movement. The exercises will include the vestibular moves that use the eyes and head in various manners as well as larger movements that include standing and walking exercises. Doing the eye and brain exercises first allows you to stop and recover from any dizziness before embarking on the larger movements required in the standing and walking ones.

Day 1
- o   Eyes Side-to-Side (Ch. 6)
- o   Eyes Up and Down (Ch. 6)
- o   Single Leg Stance (Ch. 3)
- o   Lateral Stepping (Ch. 3)

Day 2
- o   Gaze Stabilization Sitting (Ch. 6)
- o   Smooth Pursuits (Ch. 6)
- o   Trunk Circles (Ch. 2)
- o   Tandem Stance (Ch. 3)

72

Day 3

- ○ Head and Eyes Same Direction (Ch. 6)
- ○ Head and Eyes Opposite Direction (Ch. 6)
- ○ Narrow Stance Reach (Ch. 3)
- ○ Standing Marches (Ch. 3)

Day 4

- ○ Head Bend (Ch. 6)
- ○ Head Turn (Ch. 6)
- ○ Mini Lunges (Ch. 3)
- ○ Heel-to-Toe (Ch. 4)

Day 5

- ○ Shoulder Turns (Ch. 6)
- ○ Gaze Stabilization Standing (Ch. 6)
- ○ Sit-to-Stand (Ch. 2)
- ○ Foot Taps (Ch. 3)

WALKING AND MOVEMENT WEEK

Working on your balance while walking requires you to do several things at the same time. Before attempting this week's routine, be sure that you are at a comfortable level in your stability and are able to do all the seated, standing, core, and vestibular exercises.

Day 1

- ○ Hip External Rotator Stretch (Ch. 2)
- ○ Grapevine (Ch. 4)
- ○ 3-Way Hip Kick (Ch. 3)
- ○ Dynamic Walking (Ch. 4)

Day 2

- ○ Squats (Ch. 3)
- ○ Walk on Heels and Tiptoes (Ch. 4)
- ○ Standing Marches (Ch. 3)
- ○ Side Steps (Ch. 4)

Day 3

- ○ Heel Raises (Ch. 3)
- ○ Balance Walk (Ch. 4)
- ○ Heel-to-Toe (Ch. 4)
- ○ Ball Toss (Ch. 4)

Day 4

- ○ Seated Forward Roll Ups (Ch. 5)
- ○ Curb Walk (Ch. 4)
- ○ Grapevine (Ch. 4)
- ○ Backward Walking (Ch. 4)

Day 5

- ○ Seated Side Bends (Ch. 5)
- ○ Dynamic Walking (Ch. 4)
- ○ Side Steps (Ch. 4)
- ○ Zigzag Walk (Ch. 4)

Conclusion

We can't avoid age. However, we can avoid some aging. Continue to do things. Be active. Life is fantastic in the way it adjusts to demands; if you use your muscles and mind, they stay there much longer.

—Charles H. Townes

Well done, reader, on taking the initiative to regain and maintain your balance! By being your own advocate for healthy living and wellness maintenance, you have taken charge of your body and its well being. As we learned throughout the book, there are many things we can do to help our bodies remain strong and stable even as we get older. Aging doesn't have to mean fading, health-wise. Remaining active and engaging in regular physical activity can result in longevity, adding years to your life. Equally important, however, is that by continuing to exercise and be active, you are adding life to your remaining years.

We learned early on in the book that by keeping a regular exercise routine, we can accomplish things like:

o   Helping prevent illness and disease

o   Encouraging good mental health

o   Improving cognitive functioning

o   Lessening the risk of falling

o   Staying connected with others

Older adults can hold many misconceptions about exercise, including thoughts of being too old or too weak. The reality is that exercise is what keeps us youthful in mind and spirit, helps ward off illness and chronic disease, and maintains our weight and balance in the long run. By including exercise in the key four areas of cardiovascular, strength training, flexibility, and balance, we can stay healthy and productive for the remainder of our lives. We learned that exercise doesn't have to be strenuous or hard to be effective, which is good news especially for those with medical problems or limited mobility. Any kind of movement is good for the body.

In learning about how our body regulates balance, we saw that there are many layers to everything in our body working together. The sensory information that we get from our eyes, ears, skin, muscles, and joints all get sent to the the brain, which then processes that input. After integrating all the bits and pieces of information, the brain sends messages to the rest of the body, including the arms, legs, feet, and core, as to what responses to make, or what things to adjust, to keep everything stable.

Next, we looked at the reality and consequences of falling because of the loss of balance. The data on the fall rates of those over 65 years old shows that a quarter of the older population falls every year and will continue to experience falls after the initial one. The consequences of falling can be serious injury to the brain, broken bones, internal bleeding, and potentially the loss of independence because of the fall outcome. Many factors contribute to the fall risk factors including: reduced or poor vision, foot problems, medication side-effects, vitamin D deficiency, and tripping hazards in the home. Preventative measures can be taken to reduce the likelihood of tripping and falling, such as getting an eye exam, checking with your doctor about your medications and vitamin D supplements, and making needed changes in your home to reduce the risk of falls.

The balance test at the end of Chapter 1 gave us an idea of how robust our balance was currently and the following chapters outlined how we can effectively boost our body's ability to remain stable while sitting, standing, and walking.

The balance exercises we learned in this book comprised of:

○ **Seated exercises.** The 10 exercises in this chapter concentrated on simple movements to train and retrain our muscles for stability from a seated position.

○ **Standing exercises.** Progressing to a standing position, we worked on specific exercises that mimic everyday activities and tasks while building balance on our feet.

○ **Walking exercises.** These exercises incorporated movement in the standing position and had us moving in small and big ways as our body practiced it's balance while walking.

○ **Core exercises.** Because our core muscles, those in our abdomen, back, and glutes, hold our body upright, we worked on strengthening our core in ways that are back- and neck-friendly.

○ **Vestibular exercises.** The last type of exercises concentrated on our eyes, ears, and brain, also known as the vestibular system. A stable vestibular system is key to good balance and control.

Lastly, we talked about how to implement all that we have learned in this book into a daily program. Depending on your goals, you can choose to incorporate the exercises into your fitness routine in a variety of ways. Adding in one exercise a day is a simple way to get started and allows you to methodically work through each exercise until you complete all fifty. Another option was to implement the exercises on a chapter-by-chapter basis. For those looking for a plug and play program, we looked at a month's worth of balance exercise routines that outline a weekly and daily schedule of what to do.

My hope and desire is that you have benefitted not only from the information and encouragement in this book, but that you also make these exercises a part of your daily life in regaining and maintaining your balance.

SCAN THE QR CODE

I trust you will experience excellent health and well-being on the long road of life that lies before you and wish you my very best. Thank you for letting me share my knowledge with you.

Baz Thompson

References

16 positive quotes about ageing. (2019, May 9). Brightwatergroup.com. https://brightwatergroup.com/news-articles/16-positive-quotes-about-ageing/

Akdeniz, S., Hepguler, S., Öztürk, C., & Atamaz, F. C. (2016). The relation between vitamin D and postural balance according to clinical tests and tetrax posturography. *Journal of Physical Therapy Science, 28*(4), 1272–1277. https://doi.org/10.1589/jpts.28.1272

Baker, J. (2020, October 19). *Why you need to test your balance (plus 3 exercises to improve it).* Whole Life Challenge. https://www.wholelifechallenge.com/why-you-need-to-test-your-balance-plus-3-exercises-to-improve-it/

Balance exercises for stroke patients: How to improve stability. (2020, June 3). Flint Rehab. https://www.flintrehab.com/balance-exercises-for-stroke-patients/

Balance tests: MedlinePlus lab test information. (2019). Medlineplus.gov. https://medlineplus.gov/lab-tests/balance-tests/

Bedosky, L. (2021, March 13). *The best core exercises for seniors.* Get Healthy U | Chris Freytag. https://gethealthyu.com/best-core-exercises-for-seniors/

Betty Friedan quotes. (n.d.). BrainyQuote. https://www.brainyquote.com/quotes/betty_friedan_383994?src=t_aging

Bumgardner, W. (2020, May 29). *10 fun ways to add balance exercises to your walks.* Verywell Fit. https://www.verywellfit.com/add-balance-exercises-to-your-walks-4142274

CDC. (2019a). *Important facts about falls.* Cdc.gov. https://www.cdc.gov/homeandrecreationalsafety/falls/adultfalls.html

CDC. (2019b). *Older adults: Physical activity and health. Surgeon General report.* Centers for Disease Control and Prevention. https://www.cdc.gov/nccdphp/sgr/olderad.htm

Centers for Disease Control. (n.d.). *What you can do to prevent falls.* https://www.cdc.gov/steadi/pdf/STEADI-Brochure-WhatYouCanDo-508.pdf

Charles H. Townes quotes. (n.d.). BrainyQuote. Retrieved November 6, 2021, from https://www.brainyquote.com/quotes/charles_h_townes_639625?src=t_aging

Continued vestibular rehabilitation exercises -level 1 general information for eye exercises. (n.d.). https://ahc.aurorahealthcare.org/fywb/x20521.pdf

David Linley quotes. (n.d.). BrainyQuote. Retrieved November 6, 2021, from https://www.brainyquote.com/quotes/david_linley_1145134

Eartha Kitt quotes. (n.d.). BrainyQuote. Retrieved November 6, 2021, from https://www.brainyquote.com/quotes/eartha_kitt_474182

Elsawy, B., & Higgins, K. E. (2010). Physical activity guidelines for older adults. *American Family Physician*, *81*(1), 55–59. https://www.aafp.org/afp/2010/0101/p55.html

Fratacelli, T. (2019, May 19). *12 balance exercises for seniors | with printable pictures and PDF.* PTProgress | Career Development, Education, Health. https://www.ptprogress.com/balance-exercises-for-seniors/

George Burns quotes. (n.d.). BrainyQuote. Retrieved November 6, 2021, from https://www.brainyquote.com/quotes/george_burns_103932?src=t_getting_older

Gottberg, K. (2016, November 4). *50 of the best positive aging quotes I could find.* SMART Living 365. https://www.smartliving365.com/50-best-positive-aging-quotes-find/

Hoffman, H. (2017, July 18). *5 best sitting balance exercises for stroke patients (with videos) | saebo.* Saebo. https://www.saebo.com/blog/5-best-sitting-balance-exercises-stroke-patients-videos/

Peter Diamandis quotes. (n.d.). BrainyQuote. Retrieved November 6, 2021, from https://www.brainyquote.com/quotes/peter_diamandis_690491

Robinson, L. (2019). *Senior exercise and fitness tips*. HelpGuide.org. https://www.helpguide.org/articles/healthy-living/exercise-and-fitness-as-you-age.htm

Schrift, D. (2019). *12 best elderly balance exercises for seniors to reduce the risk of falls*. Eldergym® Senior Fitness. https://eldergym.com/elderly-balance/

The best core exercises for older adults. (2021, April 1). Harvard Health. https://www.health.harvard.edu/staying-healthy/the-best-core-exercises-for-older-adults

The GreenFields. (2016). *5 benefits of exercise for seniors and aging adults | the greenfields continuing care community | lancaster, NY*. Thegreenfields.org. https://thegreenfields.org/5-benefits-exercise-seniors-aging-adults/

Vestibular_Exercises. (n.d.). University of Mississippi Medical Center. Retrieved October 27, 2021, from https://www.umc.edu/Healthcare/ENT/Patient-Handouts/Adult/Otology/Vestibular_Exercises.html

Villines, Z. (2020, October 20). *Balance problems: Symptoms, diagnosis, and treatment*. Www.medicalnewstoday.com. https://www.medicalnewstoday.com/articles/balance-problems#when-to-see-a-doctor

Watson, M. A., Black, F. O., & Crowson, M. (n.d.). *The human balance system*. VeDA. https://vestibular.org/article/what-is-vestibular/the-human-balance-system/the-human-balance-system-how-do-we-maintain-our-balance/

Printed in the USA
CPSIA information can be obtained
at www.ICGtesting.com
LVHW080901101123
763411LV00030B/38